Inspired Journal

A Companion to Inspired Nurse

Rich Bluni, RN

All rights reserved.
Published by:
Fire Starter Publishing
913 Gulf Breeze Parkway, Suite 6
Gulf Breeze, FL 32561
Phone: 850-934-1099
Fax: 850-934-1384
www.firestarterpublishing.com

ISBN: 978-0-9749986-9-5

Library of Congress Control Number: 2009921427

Printed in the United States of America

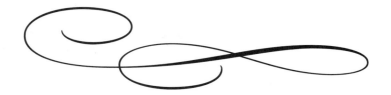

TABLE OF CONTENTS

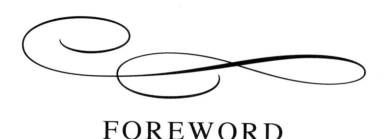

FOREWORD

A WORD FROM QUINT STUDER

Never underestimate the difference one person can make.

As I travel the country, I hear many inspiring stories about the impact people in healthcare have on others.

A healthcare professional might offer therapeutic touch, a word of compassion, or an easy-to-grasp explanation of a complicated diagnosis. Whether they realize it at the time or not, nurses, doctors, and other care providers make a real difference in patients' lives.

One of my favorite stories involves a nurse who went to her son's kindergarten open house. As she was perched on his small chair, a woman sat beside her and said, "I have your photo in my wallet."

Noticing the nurse's bewildered expression, the woman explained that her son was born in extremely critical condition and spent time in the NICU. She had been so terrified that he would not make it. Wanting to at least have a photo of her precious child, she asked the nurse to hold her baby so she could take a picture.

The good news is that the little boy survived and years later ended up in the same kindergarten class as the son of the nurse who held him for his first photo! Instead of the baby picture many mothers keep with them, this woman carried a photo of a NICU nurse holding her son. And now, coincidentally, the two mothers found themselves sitting across from each other at their boys' school.

Nurses inspire others through their selfless devotion. Our research on women and work-life blend shows that while nurses take wonderful care of their patients, they sometimes sacrifice their own well-being in the process. (See page 95 for a summary of Studer Group's study titled *Work-Life Blend among Women in the Healthcare Industry*.)

Nurses must frequently make tough decisions between spending time at work (for the good of patients) and at home (for the good of their families and themselves). That is why Studer Group's goal is to help nurses be as efficient as possible so that they can more effectively manage this pull between their professional and personal lives.

Our study showed that nurses feel comfortable doing something for themselves only two times per year. And when they do take the rare moment for themselves, they often experience guilt about what they are not doing for others during this time.

We hope *Inspired Journal*, along with its companion book, *Inspired Nurse* (written by Studer Group's own Rich Bluni, RN), will change that mindset. Together, they can help nurses take time to reflect on themselves and the difference they make in others' lives—and remind them to do what they can to take care of themselves.

What are you doing to be good to you? Perhaps *Inspired Journal* can help you answer that question for yourself. And perhaps it can help your colleagues and coworkers answer that question, too.

Nurses deserve to be taken care of, both as a profession and as individuals. One inspired nurse can make a huge difference in the lives of those he or she touches. And an organization filled with them is an unstoppable force for good.

Quint Studer

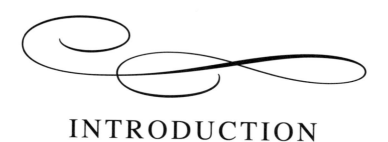

INTRODUCTION

YOUR JOURNEY TO INSPIRATION BEGINS HERE.

I believe it was E.M. Forster who said, "How do I know what I think until I see what I say?" I love that quote. To me, it expresses what makes journaling so powerful.

There is something truly magical about putting pen to paper—something that helps you unearth and articulate your deepest, most secret thoughts and feelings.

And if you're a nurse seeking to rediscover (or hold onto) the sense of inspiration with which you began your career, journaling can transform your life. It can unleash amazing spiritual and emotional growth.

Inspired Journal is designed to be a companion to my book *Inspired Nurse*. Each section in this journal corresponds to one of the book's chapters, beginning with an excerpt (sometimes lightly embellished) from the "Inspiration Destination" that follows each of my personal stories.

Please use this journal in the way that works best for you. You might do your writing alongside your reading of *Inspired Nurse*, one chapter at a time. Or you might wait until you've read the entire book to begin journaling. If you run out of pages, you might choose to continue in a notebook or perhaps on the computer.

This is your journal—and your journey. Thank you for letting me be a part of it.

Rich Bluni, RN
Author of *Inspired Nurse*

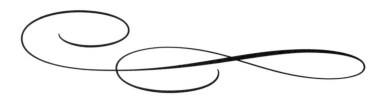

COMPANION READING:
Inspired Nurse Chapter 1

INSPIRATION DESTINATION: TEN MINUTES OF PURPOSE.

Carve out ten minutes. During this time, think about an occasion when you felt you made a difference as a nurse—one in which you felt connected to your purpose. Perhaps think of this moment as your "most inspiring nursing experience ever."

Close your eyes and relive that experience. Remember the sounds and the sights. Hear the voices. Hear the monitor bells; see the defibrillator reach its charge. Get back there. Your goal is to recreate the whole experience for yourself.

Embrace the feeling of purpose. Feel the sense of pride, of accomplishment. Now, journal your inspiration. Write about this experience. Write about others you've had.

Write the "good" stories. They may not have had happy endings, but perhaps they opened your eyes or motivated you to be better. Such moments make all the difference.

Think about these pivotal times in your work. Are there days where inspiration is right in front of you? What does the following sentence mean to you: *Look for reasons to be inspired.*

Chapter 1

Inspired Journal

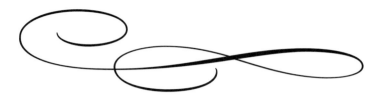

COMPANION READING:
Inspired Nurse Chapter 2

INSPIRATION DESTINATION: HONOR YOUR MENTOR.

Who first suggested nursing school to you? Who did you cry to during your exams? Who was your best preceptor? Who was that manager who insisted, "You can do this!" when you thought for sure that you could not? Who was that nursing instructor who amazed you with her combination of heart, brains, and caring? Who was that experienced nurse who took you under her wing and showed you the ropes?

Think where you would be without any one of these people. Imagine how much more difficult your job would be without the foundation that they helped create. Honor them by telling them "thank you"...and by writing about the gifts they've shared with you.

Honoring mentors reminds you that there are people along the way who have made this journey possible, meaningful, and even beautiful. You are here today because of them.

Write the qualities, in single adjectives, that describe one of your mentors. They may be "honest" or "smart" or "empathetic." Think about what these words mean to you in your journey as a nurse. What have you learned from your mentor that you can use to mentor others?

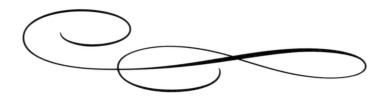

Chapter 2

COMPANION READING:
Inspired Nurse Chapter 3

INSPIRATION DESTINATION: THANK A FAMILY MEMBER OR FRIEND FOR HIS OR HER SUPPORT.

What family member, significant other, or friend has been a key to your nursing success? Maybe a sibling babysat your kids so you could attend class? Maybe your mom brought dinner to your dorm room? Maybe your dad "loaned" you the money for nursing school and then as a graduation gift told you not to worry about paying him back? Maybe your friend drove you to school in the morning?

Few of us took this journey without anyone's help. Think about someone who offered you support. Send her a thank-you note, call her, or bring her flowers. Then, write about this experience.

The inspiration does not solely lie in your loved one's reaction or in making her feel good. It dwells in the act of giving gratitude and reverence to someone who helped make it possible for you to touch all of the lives you have touched and will touch as a nurse.

What would you like to tell others who nurtured you? Journal your message to them and the impact they have had on you. Perhaps you'll decide to share it with them. Perhaps not. Either way, the gratitude you feel will nourish your own spirit.

Chapter 3

Purpose,
worthwhile work
and making
a difference

PRINCIPLES

PILLAR RESULTS

PASSION

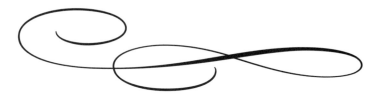

COMPANION READING:
Inspired Nurse Chapter 4

INSPIRATION DESTINATION: SUPPORT NEW NURSES.

Think back to when you were "the new nurse." It was surely a challenge. Being the new *anything* can be a challenge. It seems everyone knows everything already, and the simplest tasks take you five times longer than they do everyone else.

Remember looking around for that friendly face, kind smile, and patient voice? When you found that, it was a place of rest, a sanctuary from the fear and self-doubt that you sometimes felt would smother you. Journal your thoughts on those first days as a nurse.

Can you find a way to smooth the path for some other new kid on the block? Who knows what that simple gesture may bring to harvest in the future.

Ask yourself, *What three things do I wish someone would have said to or done for me when I was just starting out?* Write them down here.

Chapter 4

Purpose,
worthwhile work
and making
a difference

PRINCIPLES
PILLAR RESULTS
PASSION

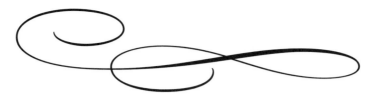

COMPANION READING:
Inspired Nurse Chapter 5

INSPIRATION DESTINATION: NOTICE THE MIRACULOUS.

During your time as a nurse, have you experienced something that you can't explain? An amazing recovery? A healing that left the team scratching their heads in disbelief?

If you haven't yet experienced that personally, do you know of someone who has? What was his or her story? Maybe in your life outside of work you have been witness to something "miraculous" or have a family story that has been passed down to you. Where has the miraculous touched your life?

If it is a story you recall, write it down. If it is something that you are hoping for, whether it's for a patient or a friend, journal about it. Perhaps start off by writing "I define a miracle as..." and then take it from there.

Journal about the miracle you were part of. Journal about the miracle you heard about. Journal about the miracle that you would like to see happen. It is inspirational to connect to the "miraculous"...whatever that means to you.

Chapter 5

PRINCIPLES

PILLAR RESULTS

Purpose,
worthwhile work
and making
a difference

PASSION

®

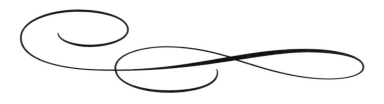

COMPANION READING:

Inspired Nurse Chapter 6

INSPIRATION DESTINATION: GIVE GRATITUDE TO NURSING AIDES/ASSISTANTS.

No matter what you do in nursing, someone is there supporting your work. If you are a nursing executive, you may have an assistant, a staff nurse may have nursing aides, a professor may have a teaching assistant, a researcher may have a data processor.

Choose one of your most helpful assistants and let her know that her support is priceless. The method is not nearly as important as the intent. Your goal is simple. Give your gratitude to someone who supports your work. Be specific. Let her know exactly what she does that makes such a difference to you.

Write about how it feels to give this gift of gratitude. What did you see or hear from the one you shared with? What feels different? Would you do it again? Why or why not? If someone recognized you in this way, how would you want them to do so?

Chapter 6

PRINCIPLES

PILLAR RESULTS

Purpose,
worthwhile work
and making
a difference

PASSION

®

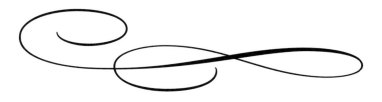

COMPANION READING:
Inspired Nurse Chapter 7

INSPIRATION DESTINATION: MAKE YOUR WORKPLACE MORE PEACEFUL.

The nursing environment can sometimes "breed" manic energy. For contrast, think about a bookstore, a house of worship, or a library. Few people walk into these places yelling or talking loudly or fussing. Yet, most of us have seen our peers and coworkers do such things in our own workplace.

Ask yourself, *Is my personal or shared workspace peaceful? Is there anything I can do to make it more peaceful?* Your workspace may be a busy ER, a clinic, an office, a classroom, a skills lab, an ICU, a nursing unit, or any number of other places. So be creative. What can you do to bring peace to your environment?

Journal your ideas. What might your peaceful new workspace feel like? Look like? Sound like? How would it impact you and those around you?

Chapter 7

Purpose,
worthwhile work
and making
a difference

PRINCIPLES

PILLAR RESULTS

PASSION

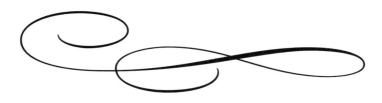

COMPANION READING:
Inspired Nurse Chapter 8

INSPIRATION DESTINATION: WRITE A THANK-YOU NOTE.

Thank-you notes are powerful things. They take a feeling or thought of appreciation and turn it into something tangible. You can hold them, read and re-read them, and share them with others.

Think of someone who has made a difference in your life. It could be a coworker, a friend, or even someone who gave you great service in a store or restaurant. Write him or her a thank-you note. Then, journal about how this gesture made you feel. What was his or her response?

You might also journal about a time you received a heartfelt thank-you note. How did it feel to be so appreciated? Did it inspire you to be even more helpful or giving in the future?

Purpose, worthwhile work and making a difference

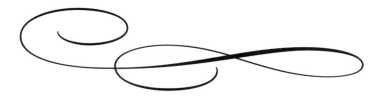

COMPANION READING:

Inspired Nurse Chapter 9

INSPIRATION DESTINATION: ASK A PATIENT OR COWORKER FOR HIS OR HER "ONE THING."

Hold up the mirror. What do you see? Are you asking those that you serve, "What can I do for you?" or are you asking, "What can you do for me?" How do you think others perceive you? Is your mirror so fogged up from speaking about yourself that you can't see those standing behind you who really need your support?

Ask a patient, "If there was one thing that I could do for you today to make you feel a little better, what would that one thing be?" Listen to him closely. He may not understand the question. Ask it again.

If you are no longer in patient care, adjust this practice to fit your own life. Perhaps you'll decide to ask a coworker the "one thing" question.

Your goal here is simple. Find something that you can do for this person to bring him some comfort or support. You will find in that simple act a surprising sense of inspiration.

What was the reaction to your question? Journal about it. Did you find the "one thing" to be simple or complex? How did this process impact you?

Purpose,
worthwhile work
and making
a difference

PRINCIPLES

PILLAR RESULTS

PASSION

®

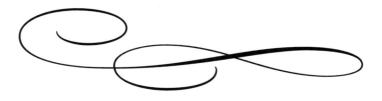

COMPANION READING:
Inspired Nurse Chapter 10

INSPIRATION DESTINATION: BE WELCOMING OF SPIRIT.

Many of us find peace in spirit. Some of us may have a deep relationship with God, others may have a spiritual knowing, still others may have neither. It is what it is.

Personal beliefs aside, are there times when you can be a part of the peace your patients may find in their spiritual walk? Is there a way that you can feed this need that your patients may have?

If your patient has a need for a spiritual boost, maybe you can simply offer to wheel him down to the chapel on your break, or buy him a book he indicated he might like, or arrange to have members of his place of worship gather with him. If you don't feel like you can be a participant, can you find ways to be an agent?

How can you make spirit a part of your inspired journey? And if you are a "spiritual rebel" how can you help a patient with his or her spiritual needs? Explore your thoughts in this journal.

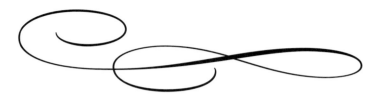

Chapter 10

COMPANION READING:
Inspired Nurse Chapter 11

INSPIRATION DESTINATION: INCREASE AND IMPROVE PATIENT SAFETY.

Medical errors happen. And when we hear about them—or worse, are involved in one—we are drained of inspiration. We healthcare professionals are the "second victims" when errors occur. Each of us carries the burden of errors committed, either by us personally or by our team or organization.

On the other hand, we gain inspiration when we know that we have protected our patients and ensured that their care was safe.

Journal about errors you have made. Choose to not dwell on what went wrong but rather on how you can prevent it from happening again.

What ideas do you have? How can you learn and grow from your mistakes? What can you do to increase and improve patient safety?

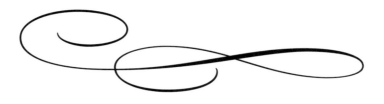

Chapter 11

COMPANION READING:
Inspired Nurse Chapter 12

INSPIRATION DESTINATION: SEEK THE GOOD IN OTHERS.

Your challenge is simple: Look for something good in each person you encounter today, whether they're coworkers, friends, employees, or strangers you pass in the hallway.

Hopefully, you will recognize that we each *decide* that someone is "bad" or "stupid" or "fun" or "wonderful." Why not decide to look for the good rather than the bad or the ugly? And if you can do it for one day, might you be able to do it every day?

Start looking for opportunities to be encouraged and impressed and inspired. You will find that this opens your heart for more inspiration.

Journal what it was like to spend a day looking for the good in people. Once you become more practiced at it, does it become easier? How has it changed your relationships? How has it changed *you*?

Purpose, worthwhile work and making a difference

PRINCIPLES

PILLAR RESULTS

PASSION

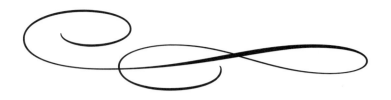

COMPANION READING:
Inspired Nurse Chapter 13

INSPIRATION DESTINATION: LOOK FOR REASONS TO BE INSPIRED.

You have one goal today. Be "present" in all that you do. Listen for words that inspire you. Look for deeds that inspire you. Prepare yourself to hear stories that will inspire you. It is a funny truth that when you look for something, or introduce something into your awareness, it suddenly becomes evident everywhere.

What if you challenged yourself to become aware of inspiration? What if this became a habit? You often see the opposite. People look for reasons to be insulted or outraged and they are never disappointed, are they? Why not do the opposite? Why not look for reasons to be inspired instead?

What did you learn? Ponder the lesson. Was the inspiration you encountered something new...or something that you simply did not see before? Can you do this on subsequent days? What if you tried it at home?

This is where your journal comes in handy. Write down your experiences. They become tangible for you when you can revisit them. It is awe-inspiring when you become aware of all of the inspiration in your world.

Chapter 13

PRINCIPLES
PILLAR RESULTS
PASSION

Purpose,
worthwhile work
and making
a difference

®

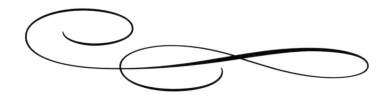

COMPANION READING:
Inspired Nurse Chapter 14

INSPIRATION DESTINATION: SHARE YOUR STORIES.

Think about the stories your parents told you. If you were fortunate enough to have had a relationship with grandparents or even great-grandparents, do you remember the stories they would tell? Our history allows us to reflect, refresh, and learn. Our stories make our experiences tangible. Stories allow us to hold our reality in our hands. Tell your stories.

What is the toughest thing you can ever recall having dealt with during your healthcare journey? Was it a person? A natural or man-made disaster? How did it change you? How did it change your life perspective? Did you almost throw in the professional towel?

Now what's the funniest thing that has ever happened to you? The most absurd situation you have ever been in? It's okay if it is a little "out there." It's good to laugh.

Your journal is crying out to you right now. Write your stories down. Take your time. Throw yourself into it, or if you're inclined, video yourself telling your stories. Then read/watch your storytelling. Cry. Laugh. Remember.

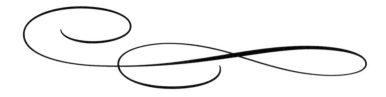

Chapter 14

COMPANION READING:
Inspired Nurse Chapter 15

INSPIRATION DESTINATION: APPRECIATE HUMOR.

What so often sustains us is humor. It has rescued the soul of many a person. Think about how good laughter is for you. It heals, elevates, refreshes.

Using your journal, write down what you think is funny. Who is your favorite comedic actor or actress? What movies make you laugh? Who is the funniest person you know? Who makes you laugh at work? Who always has a funny joke to tell, an embarrassing story, or great witty comebacks? Is it you? Ponder what laughter means to you.

We have two choices in life. We laugh or we cry. Sometimes we laugh so hard that we cry; sometimes we cry so much we eventually start to laugh at how ridiculous the situation is. Share a time when humor has helped you make it through a tough nursing day.

Knowing that laughter and tears are often interchangeable, write about how you can choose laughter. Do you take yourself so seriously that you've become rigid? How can you make humor a mainstay?

Purpose, worthwhile work and making a difference

PRINCIPLES

PILLAR RESULTS

PASSION

®

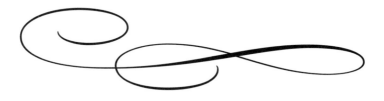

COMPANION READING:
Inspired Nurse Chapter 16

INSPIRATION DESTINATION: SHARE THE INSPIRATION. INSPIRE IT FORWARD.

SPIRITUAL STRETCH #1: What if there is good inside you and it only ever stays there? If there is music in your heart, or laughter in your spirit, who does it help if it always stays hidden? Remember the parable about the lantern kept under a bushel. If its light is hidden, to whom does it show the way? Get it?

So, if you feel a sense of inspiration, *inspire it forward*. Who comes to mind that could use a boost in spirit? Do you work with anyone who once had that glowing spirit and through life circumstance, or work stressors, lost it?

Tell her exactly what it is about her you find inspiring—her assessment skills, for example, or her ability to run a meeting, or her willingness to help others.

Journal about how this person reacted. What did she say? How did her body language change? How did it impact her? How did it impact you?

Chapter 16

PRINCIPLES

PILLAR RESULTS

Purpose,
worthwhile work
and making
a difference

PASSION

®

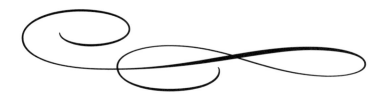

COMPANION READING:
Inspired Nurse Chapter 17

INSPIRATION DESTINATION: PERFORM AN ANONYMOUS ACT OF KINDNESS.

Do something nice for someone without letting her know you did it. Why does your act of kindness have to be anonymous? Because the inspiration is not in getting a thank you, but in the simple act of the kindness. That's it. You will walk away feeling as if you and the universe share some sweet, beautiful secret.

It is inspiring to make a difference. It is inspiring to help. It is inspiring to be in it for nothing more than to be in it. There is such a powerful energy in the act of giving. Why *is* that, do you think?

Ask yourself that question. Journal about it.

This is your journey. How do you give? In what ways do you find inspiration in giving? Is it easy or hard for you to be anonymous when you give? Learn about yourself. Dig deeper. Really chew on this for a while. What can you discover about yourself and inspiration as it relates to giving?

Purpose,
worthwhile work
and making
a difference

PRINCIPLES

PILLAR RESULTS

PASSION

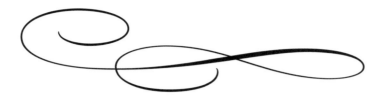

COMPANION READING:

Inspired Nurse Chapter 18

INSPIRATION DESTINATION: GIVE OF YOUR TIME AND KNOWLEDGE.

Often the best way to connect to your passion is to give of yourself and your time. What better way is there to be inspired than to see the appreciation in the eyes of someone you have helped, for no other reason than because you cared? Not as part of your job, or for pay, or even for a pat on the back...just because.

Giving of your time and expertise serves the dual purpose of inspiring self and inspiring others. The caring heart that you possess as a nurse needs to be fed. Not doing so deprives you of the fuel you need to sustain your spirit in this field.

Maybe you already are volunteering or mentoring. If not, there must be some way you can give back. And while you may not be able to start your volunteer work today, you *can* plan it, look for it, talk about it with your peers or friends, ask questions, journal about it, inquire about it, and put the wheels in motion.

Write about the impact volunteering has had on those you have helped. Even more important, how has it impacted you? Have you become kinder? More generous? Less judgmental and more forgiving? What has giving taught you about yourself?

Purpose,
worthwhile work
and making
a difference

PRINCIPLES

PILLAR RESULTS

PASSION

®

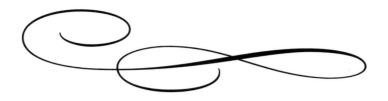

COMPANION READING:
Inspired Nurse Chapter 19

INSPIRATION DESTINATION: MAKE A WHY-I'M-GRATEFUL-FOR-BEING-A-NURSE LIST.

You've probably heard about gratitude lists before. Well, now is the time to make one. But give it a different spin: Focus on what you are most grateful for as it relates to being a nurse.

What do you love about being a nurse? What are the best parts? What keeps you going? What does a good day look like? How has being a nurse made you a better human being?

Start off the list by writing, "As a nurse I am very grateful for..." and then go at it.

There are many great things about being a nurse. You know that already. Making a list will help you remember it.

Purpose,
worthwhile work
and making
a difference

PRINCIPLES

PILLAR RESULTS

PASSION

®

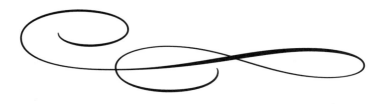

COMPANION READING:
Inspired Nurse Chapter 20

INSPIRATION DESTINATION: WATCH YOUR MOUTH! (USE NEW WORDS.)

Words are powerful things. They heal nations. They change lives. They can change yours—for better or for worse.

What words do you use on a regular basis? Do you use words like "fried," "burnt," "tired," "overworked," "stressed," and the like? You can *hear* yourself. You can also *heal* yourself.

What you say influences how you feel. You may have heard it called "self-talk." Today, speak the language of inspiration. Use phrases and words that have that feel to them: "good," "great," "wonderful," "smart," "love."

Journal about your day or your patients or your coworkers or your last shift...but make this entry positive. How do the words on the page make you feel? What kind of power do they project?

Purpose, worthwhile work and making a difference

PRINCIPLES
PILLAR RESULTS
PASSION

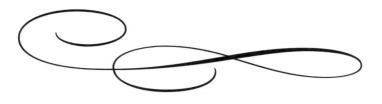

COMPANION READING:

Inspired Nurse Chapter 21

INSPIRATION DESTINATION: CREATE AFFIRMATIONS AND USE THEM TO CHANGE YOUR LIFE.

Affirmations are purposeful self-talk in which you affirm a positive outlook or outcome for your life. When you do this on a regular basis, it feeds your mind.

Think about what you want to change or improve. This can be personal or nursing-related, but as you are on the journey for inspiration in your nursing life, make at least a few affirmations specific to that. You may want to feel healthier, more confident, more in touch with Spirit. You may want to be more caring, improve your work or personal relationships, or have an overall more positive outlook. What do you want to affect for the better? How can you be more inspired?

Write your affirmations in your journal. Then, read back through them. How did this process make you feel?

Consciously feel and see what you are saying. Make these words real. If you are speaking about peace, then see peace in your mind and feel peace in your body. If you are speaking about health, then feel healthy. See and feel yourself feeling good, strong, confident, in shape, or whatever "healthy" means to you. Align your words, your mind, and your senses.

Purpose,
worthwhile work
and making
a difference

PRINCIPLES

PILLAR RESULTS

PASSION

®

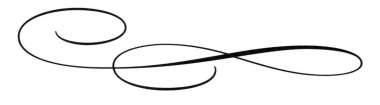

COMPANION READING:
Inspired Nurse Chapter 22

INSPIRATION DESTINATION: MAKE AN INSPIRATION PLAN.

Becoming more inspired won't be something that you stumble upon or luck into. You can't read *Inspired Nurse*, or go to a seminar, or find a four-leaf clover and hope for inspiration. You need to have a plan and you need to keep your eyes on the road.

Today, make your plan. Use this journal to map it out. Decide specifically what your overall goal is. It may be "To be more inspired" or it may be "To inspire others." It may be "To feel more positive about my work, coworkers, or myself." What is your goal? Why are you reading this book?

Next, decide how you are going to measure your success. Maybe you can rate your "attitude" each day starting today on a 1-5 scale: "1" is poor and "5" is excellent as it relates to how you feel about your work and nursing. Set a goal. Make it reachable.

If you are a "1," decide that your goal is to be a "3" within, for example, 90 days. If you are a "3," strive for a "5." Of course, your ultimate goal is to be a "5" wherever you are, but you will get there. Set a goal that you can reach, and once you reach it, set another even higher.

If you don't like this system, come up with another way to measure your specific goal. Maybe track feedback from your peers or your loved ones. Maybe they can rate you. This is yours.

Next, after you have determined a goal and decided how you will measure it, decide upon the tactics that you will take to get there. Plan your tactics in increments, like 60 or 90 days. This part will be easy because you have plenty of tactics right here in this journal.

Maybe you will focus on affirmations, honoring your mentor, using different words, and ten minutes of purpose as your tactics for the first 30 days. Write this out. This is your self-evaluation. This is your road to your ultimate Inspiration Destination.

After your time frame is up, reassess where you are. Did you achieve your goal? If not, what can you do differently? If you achieved your goal, how can you either improve further or hardwire your success? Be sure to make this your own, but below is an example of what it could look like:

Goal: To feel more inspired to a level of "4" during the course of my workday within 60 days.
Measurement: Using a 1-5 scale I will evaluate my "level of inspiration" on a daily basis. 1=completely uninspired, 2=barely inspired, 3=somewhat inspired, 4=inspired, 5= very inspired.
Tactics: I will focus on 5 tactics for a 60-day period. These will be: 1. Creating affirmations. 2. Writing a daily nursing gratitude list. 3. Honoring my mentor. 4. Supporting new nurses. 5. Being welcoming of spirit.

The first part of this Inspiration Destination is about *doing*. Nothing is more practical than a step-by-step plan! This part is about *thinking*. Consider *why* you want to be more inspired.

Do you just want to "feel good"? Do you want to be authentic? Are you searching for a sense of new or regained meaning?

Also, how do you feel about this entire exercise? Are you a "planner"? Do "planning" and "goals" seem disconnected from "inspiration" for you? Why? Does it make sense to you? Why?

Journal about your feelings regarding your roadmap to a destination of inspiration. How can you get excited about this? What is in it for you? For your team? Your patients?

Chapter 22

Purpose,
worthwhile work
and making
a difference

PRINCIPLES

PILLAR RESULTS

PASSION

®

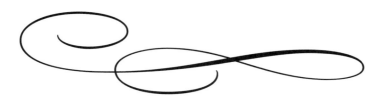

COMPANION READING:
Inspired Nurse Chapter 23

INSPIRATION DESTINATION: WRITE A LETTER FROM YOU TO YOU.

Today, write a letter in your journal. Use your imagination here. Pretend that you are writing a letter to someone you love very, very much. This person has done amazing work in her nursing career. She is deserving of hope.

You believe in this person and you want her to be uplifted. This person is your very best friend. How would you encourage her? What pearls of wisdom and inspiration could you pass along to her? What would your words of sage advice be?

This person you are writing this letter to is, of course, *you*. Take your time. Be in a place where you can be quiet. You need to really nurture this person. She needs you. Her life depends on it.

Take this seriously. What would you say to yourself if you were your own best friend? What would you want to hear from someone who loved you with all of her heart?

When you are done writing this letter, put your journal away for a couple of days. Then, revisit it. Take it to a quiet place and read your letter. Let the words sink in to your mind. They are your words, but you will notice that they somehow seem different. Appreciate the wisdom that is inside of you. You will find that you know yourself better than you thought.

That is where inspiration lives. It comes from inside—that's why it is not called "outspiration"!

Experience what it would be like to be your own best friend.

Write your letter to you.

Chapter 23

Purpose, worthwhile work and making a difference

PRINCIPLES

PILLAR RESULTS

PASSION

®

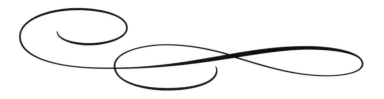

ABOUT THE AUTHOR

Rich Bluni, RN, is a national speaker and coach for Studer Group®, but the title of which he is proudest is "Nurse." An RN since 1993, he chose the profession after seeing the tremendous impact nurses had on his father after he was diagnosed with terminal cancer.

"I saw the great and small things nurses accomplished in their day and realized that there was no higher calling, for me, than to become a nurse," he says.

Rich has worked in Adolescent Oncology, Pediatric ICU, and Trauma ICU departments as well as serving as a Pedi flight and transport nurse. A Licensed Healthcare Risk Manager, he has served as ED Nursing Manager and Director of Risk Management and Patient Safety.

In 2008, he won the Studer Group Pillar Award, which is given for achievement of outstanding outcomes.

Rich and his wife, a nursing professor and former ED and Trauma nurse, live in Boynton Beach, Florida. His son Rhett is the greatest joy in his life. Today, Rich works to improve patient outcomes and encourage the spirits of nurses and all healthcare professionals who've answered the calling to serve others with their hands and hearts.

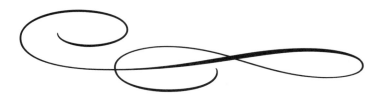

WORK-LIFE BLEND AMONG WOMEN IN THE HEALTHCARE INDUSTRY

BACKGROUND:

In 2007, Quint Studer shared a stage at a Clinical Quality Summit with Dr. Jennifer Daley, who at the time was Chief Medical Officer at Tenet Healthcare System. After the two finished presenting, they engaged the audience in a question and answer session, during which someone asked Dr. Daley not about the clinical quality or operations of the organization, but about how she balances her multiple roles in life: leader, physician, and mother. This simple question galvanized the audience that day, and sent Quint on a mission to better understand this complex and important issue. Namely, what are the unique issues that women who work in healthcare face on a daily basis? And what can their employers do to ensure that they provide the best possible place for these individuals to work?

STUDY DESIGN AND SAMPLE:

The survey consisted of a 20-minute online survey grounded in six validated work-family balance instruments. Studer Group distributed the survey nationally via healthcare associations, provider organizations, and a database of 85,000 individuals registered on www.studergroup.com.

CHARACTERISTICS OF STUDY RESPONDENTS

RESPONDENTS:

All study participants were females currently working within a healthcare provider. As a group, they are characterized as:

The largest study ever of its type -
A total of 7,792 women responded to the survey.

Geographically diverse sample –
Good representation from all regions of the US, with highest participation from the
Midwest.

Region of Residence

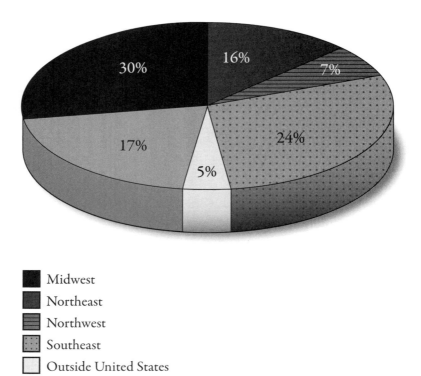

- ■ Midwest
- ■ Northeast
- ▦ Northwest
- ▦ Southeast
- ☐ Outside United States
- ■ Southwest

Representative of diverse job positions -
Including 23 percent of respondents holding positions within nursing, 22 percent in
administrative roles, 2 percent physicians and the remaining 53 percent employed in
other healthcare jobs such as therapists, non-management positions, lab personnel, etc.

Diverse Job Types

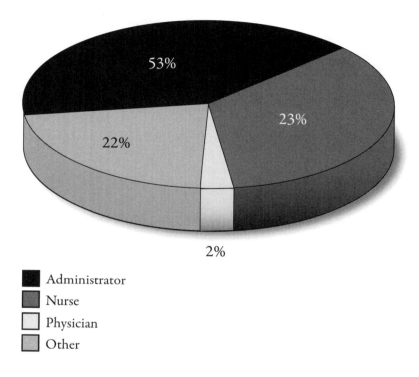

- Administrator
- Nurse
- Physician
- Other

More affluent than the general population -
Sixty-four percent have total household incomes of $75,000 or more, and 43 percent have incomes of $100,000 or more.

More than half are caregivers -
Fifty-two percent of respondents have children under 18 years of age in their household, and 23 percent have caregiving responsibilities for a dependent parent or other relative.

Work more than 40 hours each week -
For those individuals who work full-time, the average number of hours worked per week was reported as 47.7, but several worked much more: one-fourth of the respondents worked more than 50 hours per week; 10 percent of the respondents worked more than 60 hours; and 1 percent of the respondents worked 75 hours or more per week. As expected, as the number of work hours increased, individuals reported higher levels of work-life imbalance/ conflict.

Work Hours

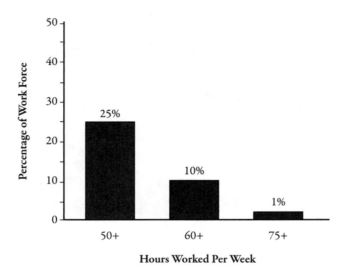

SIGNIFICANT FINDINGS

Women who responded to the study:

Would choose healthcare all over again -
More than 75 percent of respondents indicated that, if given the chance, they would choose a career in healthcare again.

Would recommend healthcare to their female friends -
Nearly 73 percent indicated that they would recommend a career in healthcare to their female friends.

Are as satisfied with their work-life as they were with their home-life -
When asked to rate their satisfaction with their work-life, 70 percent selected satisfied or very satisfied. When asked the same question about their home-life, this rating was only slightly higher at 75 percent.

Are less satisfied with the balance between their job and their home-life -
Only 47 percent are satisfied or very satisfied with their current work-life balance.

Rarely dedicate time to their personal and emotional needs -
The majority of women said they take time to treat themselves no more than once a month. Of note, 46 percent report treating themselves "rarely" (no more than a few times a year).

Experience work conflicts with home-life more frequently than home-life conflicts with work -
Forty-five percent of the respondents reported that they experienced work-family conflict at least one day or more per week. Conversely, only 6 percent noted that they experienced family interference with work at the same frequency. The following factors were associated with a higher degree of work-family conflict: individuals who worked non-dayshift and/or mandatory overtime; respondents who reported having children younger than 18 years of age in the household; individuals with caregiving responsibilities for other dependent relatives.

Find support from families and spouses -
Both spouse and family support were reported as helpful in coping with the demands of work and home. Seventy-two percent of respondents are married while the remainder are divorced and/or single, with no spousal support.

> **More than 75 percent of respondents indicated that, if given the chance, they would choose a career in healthcare again.**

IMPLICATIONS FOR EMPLOYERS

Women who responded to the study:

Use and value certain benefits more than others to help balance work and life -
Respondents were asked targeted questions regarding specific employer support strategies, including those which are currently available to them, how often they were actually used, or would be used if available.
• **Education reimbursement**
Is the most available form of employee support (82 percent) and is the most frequently used form of support (45 percent).

- **Flextime**

Is a less available form of employee support (43 percent), yet is the second most frequently used (26 percent).

- **Concierge service**

Was the most desired service that an employer could offer, with 63 percent of respondents indicating that they would use it if available. The next four most highly desired programs that would be used if available related to flexible work options: 61 percent would use a compressed work week if it were available; 52 percent would use reduced hours; 46 percent would use flextime; 40 percent would use job sharing.

Helping teach skills for time and energy management might payoff -

As compared to their female friends, respondents indicated that they have less stamina when they get home, less time for self and personal commitments, and less of a sense of balance.

Supervisors matter -

While there were significant, positive relationships between work satisfaction and reported levels of spouse support, family support, and employer support, the biggest correlation with work satisfaction was the perception of supervisor support.

Supervisors matter most- The biggest correlation with work satisfaction was the perception of supervisor support.

For more information on this study or training resources, visit www.studergroup.com/blend

This study was conducted by the StuderAlliance for Health Care Research in conjunction with Sherill Nones Cronin, PhD, RN, BC, MSN, Program Director and Professor of Nursing at the Lansing School of Nursing and Health Sciences at Bellarmine University.

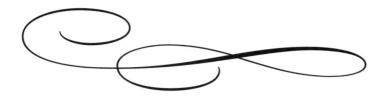

ADDITIONAL RESOURCES

Accelerate the momentum of your Healthcare Flywheel^{SM}.
Access additional resources at www.studergroup.com/inspirednurse.

Books:

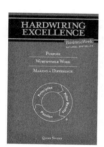

Hardwiring Excellence—In _Hardwiring Excellence_, Quint Studer helps healthcare professionals to rekindle the flame and offers a roadmap to creating and sustaining a culture of service and operational excellence that drives bottom-line results.

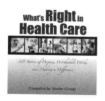

What's Right in Health Care: 365 Stories—This 742 page book shares a story a day submitted by your friends and colleagues. It is a daily reminder about why we answered this calling and why we stay with it—to serve a purpose, to do worthwhile work, and to make a difference.

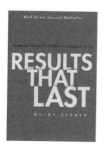

Results That Last—Healthcare leaders typically read "general business" books and figure out how to apply them to a healthcare setting. Quint's book _Results That Last_ represents a unique opportunity to share the tremendous progress our industry is making with leaders in other business arenas.

CDs:

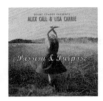 Passion & Purpose, a new CD featuring The Calling, speaks of the journey of those who are drawn to make a difference. To order, visit www.studergroup.com.

Studer Group® Institutes:

Whether your healthcare organization is just starting its journey to implementing a culture of excellence, or it is looking to create change in a specific area, Studer Group Institutes offer a range of learning opportunity.

<u>Taking You and Your Organization to the Next Level</u>—Learn the tools, tactics, and strategies that are needed to *Take You and Your Organization to the Next Level* at this two-day institute with Quint Studer and Studer Group's Coach Experts. You will walk away with Evidence-Based Leadership[SM] strategies to create a sustainable culture of execution.

<u>What's Right in Health Care</u>[SM]—One of the largest healthcare peer-to-peer learning conferences in the nation, *What's Right in Health Care* brings individuals together to share ideas that have been proven to make healthcare better.

Reignite your flame by attending any of Studer Group's passion-driven institutes. Nursing Contact Hours are awarded at each institute. Visit www.studergroup.com/institutes to view a list of upcoming institutes.

To view a list of the Nurse Contact Hours we offer for each institute, visit www.studergroup.com/CMEcredits.

Studer Group Patient Safety Toolkit:

Nothing is more foundational to our patients or to us as healthcare professionals than ensuring that patients receive safe care.

In this toolkit, we describe how specific, hardwired behaviors can be applied to patient safety. By using the same tools to improve patient safety that have already been proven to achieve clinical, operational, and service excellence, your organization will save time, expenses, and most importantly, lives. For more information on the Patient Safety Toolkit, visit www.studergroup.com.

Speakers:

Studer Group provides speaking engagements for healthcare organizations all over the country. These speakers began their lives in healthcare for many reasons, but the main reason was to make a difference in the lives of others.

Rich Bluni, RN, Studer Group National Speaker
Rich Bluni, RN, the author of *Inspired Nurse*, rates on average a *4.95 out of a 5.0* scale at his speaking engagements. Rich has more than fourteen years of clinical, legal, risk management, patient safety, and nursing management experience, and when Rich presents on stage, he brings all of his experiences to life!

To view Rich Bluni in action or to gather more information on Studer Group national speakers, visit www.studergroup.com/speakers.

Learning Videos:

AIDET^{SM} Five Fundamentals of Patient Communication
AIDET—Acknowledge, Introduce, Duration, Explanation, and Thank You—is a powerful communication tool. When interacting with patients, gaining trust is essential for obtaining patient compliance and improving clinical outcomes. AIDET is a comprehensive training tool that will enhance communication within your organization.

Hourly Rounding
Improving Nursing and Patient Care Excellence—A Studer Group Patient Care Model and video/DVD training that contains a key strategy we call hourly rounding. Hourly rounding is not only a call light reduction strategy, but also a proven tactic to reduce patient falls by 50 percent, reduce skin breakdowns by 14 percent, and improve patient satisfaction scores an average of 12 mean points.

Must Haves® Video Series
By implementing the Must Haves, healthcare organizations around the country are seeing better bottom-line results, including increased volume and decreased length of stay, as well as improved clinical outcomes, staff retention, and recruitment. The Must Haves video series consists of live lectures by Quint Studer, followed by role plays to help organizations hardwire these breakthrough practices into their culture.

Visit www.studergroup.com to view additional learning videos.

Magazines:

Hardwired Results Issue 1 Fall 2004
This issue focuses on employee loyalty. Article topics include rounding for outcomes, the power of thank you notes, a case study of Delnor Community Hospital, and a leadership self-test.

Hardwired Results Issue 7 Fall 2006
This issue features articles and tools to drive outcomes. Learn how to improve clinical outcomes with hourly rounding and increase patient satisfaction with individualized patient care.

Visit www.studergroup.com to view additional *Hardwired Results* magazines.

Webinars:

Studer Group webinars provide the latest information and tools on topics critical to healthcare leaders. Presented by Quint and other Studer Group coaches, each "on demand" webinar is an hour long. Participants will receive handouts and the opportunity to purchase the webinar on CD to teach other leaders in their organizations.

Visit www.studergroup.com to learn more about the webinars that are available.

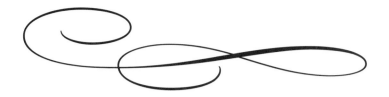

ABOUT STUDER GROUP

Studer Group is an outcomes-based healthcare consulting firm devoted to teaching evidence-based tools and processes that organizations can immediately use to create and sustain outcomes in service and operational excellence. Partner organizations see clear results in the areas of higher employee retention, greater patient and customer satisfaction, healthy financials, growing market share, and improvements in various other quality indicators. Studer Group has worked with hundreds of health care systems, hospitals, and medical groups since the firm's inception in 1999 and additionally is operating in Canada, Australia, and New Zealand.

<u>Mission and Vision</u> Studer Group's mission is to make healthcare a better place for employees to work, physicians to practice medicine, and patients to receive care. Our vision is to be the intellectual resource for healthcare professionals, combining passion with prescriptive actions and tools, to maximize human potential within each organization and healthcare as a whole.

<u>Harvesting Best Practices from a National Learning Lab</u> CEO Quint Studer and Studer Group's coaches teach, train, and speak to thousands of leaders at healthcare organizations worldwide each week, both on-site through coaching engagements and at frequent industry speaking engagements. This ongoing "in the trenches" dialogue provides ample opportunity to spot best practices in action from "first mover" innovators at many organizations. These are then harvested and tested in other organizations, refined, and shared with all healthcare organizations through peer-reviewed journal articles, Studer Group publications, and products to accelerate change.

Because we find that reducing leadership variance lies at the very heart of creating a consistent culture of excellence, Studer Group also helps organizations to hardwire great leadership. The firm retains a specialist to harvest effective tools and techniques and then share best practices for development of Leadership Development Institutes that efficiently turn training into results.

In July 2004, Studer Group also announced its Alliance for Health Care Research, which studies best practices using data from Studer Group's national learning lab to validate and quantify their impact and application at all healthcare organizations. The Alliance conducts rigorous qualitative and quantitative studies and invites participation by both client partners and non-partners of Studer Group.

<u>Resources to Support Learning</u> Studer Group's core values (teamwork, respect, integrity, generosity, and learning) are reflected in the products and services we offer. The Studer Group website, www.studergroup.com, offers a wealth of free information, articles, custom advice, and downloadable tools at no charge.

HOW TO ORDER ADDITIONAL COPIES OF

Inspired Nurse and *Inspired Journal*

Orders may be placed:

Online at:
www.firestarterpublishing.com
www.studergroup.com

By phone at: 866-354-3473

By mail at: Fire Starter Publishing
913 Gulf Breeze Parkway, Suite 6
Gulf Breeze, FL 32561

(Bulk discounts are available.)

Inspired Nurse and *Inspired Journal*
are also available online at www.amazon.com.